You deserve a smooth and acne free skin:

A simple guide on how to get rid of acne and dark spots.

Melissa Greene

Copyright
All rights reserved. No part of this publication may be reproduced, distributed, or transmitted in any form or by any means, including photocopying, recording, or other electronic or mechanical methods, without the prior written permission of the publisher, except in the case of brief quotations embodied in critical reviews and certain other noncommercial uses permitted by copyright law.

Copyright © Melissa Greene , 2023.

Contents

Introduction

Certain treatments can lessen the risk of long-haul skin difficulties like pitting and scarring. Skin inflammation imperfections fall into two classifications, contingent upon whether they cause aggravation of the encompassing skin. Most minor skin inflammation flaws are addressed by at-home consideration and non-prescription medications. Notwithstanding, individuals with extreme or long-term skin breaks ought to talk with a specialist or dermatologist. Noninflammatory skin inflammation types Whiteheads and zits are kinds of noninflammatory skin break-out sores. They are commonly the most extreme types of skin breakouts and don't cause enlargement or inconvenience. Whiteheads The clinical term for whiteheads is shut comedones. These are little, tissue-hued spots or knocks. On lighter skin, they typically have a white, round focus encompassed by a red radiance. On hazier skin, the encompassing region might seem dull or purple-tinted. Whiteheads normally don't cause scarring. The skin around a whitehead might show up close or badly crumpled, particularly when the whitehead is enormous or particularly raised. Clogged pores Clogged pores, or open comedones, are little, dull-hued detectors that might show up as somewhat raised knocks. As a rule, the skin around a pimple seems ordinary, while the focal point of the zit is hazier than the encompassing region. This hue isn't a consequence of caught soil. Clogged pores are essentially whiteheads that have opened and enlarged. At the point when the items in a whitehead are presented to air, they obscure. Treatment choices Numerous over-the-counter (OTC) flushes, lotions, gels, toners, and creams can treat noninflammatory skin breakout imperfections. They frequently contain a blend of dynamic fixes. The accompanying fixings in OTC medicines can assist with separating whiteheads and clogged pores: benzoyl peroxide salicylic corrosive azelaic corrosive adapalene A few home cures and way-of-life changes likewise can assist with diminishing generally minor-to-gentle types of noninflammatory skin break out. These include: washing with tepid water and cleanser two times a day, applying non-grating chemicals remaining hydrated trying not to over-wash or disturb the skin. restricting openness to the sun continuously wearing sunscreen when outside. Study the best sunscreen for touchy and break-out-prone skin. An individual with broken skin shouldn't disturb or pop their flaws. Doing so can prompt confusion, for example, about scarring and the arrangement of growths and knobs. Incendiary skin breakout types An individual with a more extreme instance of skin breakout may encounter excited flaws across their face, chest, and back. Incendiary skin inflammation is more serious than its noninflammatory partner and can prompt entanglements, for example, scarring and pitting. Incendiary skin inflammation can shift from little knocks that answer skin medicines to huge sores that might require careful consideration. Papules Papules are knocks under the skin's surface that are under 1 centimeter (cm) in measurement. Papules themselves will seem strong, delicate, and raised. Ordinarily, the skin around a papule is likewise kindled. Not at all like whiteheads, papules have no noticeable focus, and unlike pimples, the pores of a papule are not extended. Pustules (pimples) Pustules are bigger, delicate knocks with a characterized round community loaded up with whitish or yellowish discharge. The region around a pustule seems red or pink on a fair complexion and a profound brown or dark brown on hazier skin. The discharge in the pustule is ordinarily a mix of resistant cells and bacterial cells gathered in the impeded pore. Pustules ordinarily seem to be a lot bigger and more kindled whiteheads. Treatment choices A few home remedies and OTC medications can treat papules and pustules. These include: washing the impacted region with cool water and cleanser two times every day; utilizing items with benzoyl peroxide to battle microbes; utilizing items with salicylic corrosive to eliminate dead skin cells and other trash. A specialist can recommend different medicines, including effective dapsone and antimicrobials. Concentrates on showing that shallow synthetic face strips may likewise be a viable strategy for overseeing provocative skin break-out injuries. Extreme structures Knobs are hard, aggravated knots found profoundly inside the skin. Like papules, knobs have no apparent head. Knobs are a serious type of skin break-out imperfection and can cause skin confusion, like dim spots or scarring. This sort of skin break-out injury is created when stopped-up pores become contaminated and expand underneath the skin's surface. Therefore, nodular skin inflammation might be more serious than the actual show recommends. Growths Growths are extremely enormous, difficult, red or white bumps arranged somewhere down in the skin. Dissimilar to knobs, these pimples load up with discharge and are normally delicate to the touch. Pimples are the most serious kind of skin inflammation. In extreme cases, an individual might require careful mediation to treat them. On the off chance that not treated as expected, growths can prompt apparent scarring. Treatment choices Individuals can't generally treat extreme fiery imperfections at home. These injuries require care from a specialist or dermatologist. A specialist might suggest a blend of medications and strategies to treat knobs and sores. These may include anti-microbials, like doxycycline, and amoxicillin oral contraceptives for hormonal-related skin breakouts. efficient retinoids, for example, isotretinoin steroid infusions, photodynamic treatment to battle microbes, careful waste, and extraction to eliminate huge growths. Skin inflammation stages There are three phases of skin breakout: gentle, moderate, and extreme. The kinds of spots an individual can create during the different skin breakout stages might include: Gentle skin break out: An individual will generally develop blackheads and whiteheads in gentle skin break out. They might have a few papules and pustules. The absolute number of injuries is ordinarily under 30. Moderate skin breaks out: More papules and pustules will form when moderate skin breaks out, and an individual can likewise have a larger number of clogged pores and whiteheads. The all-out number of sores is ordinarily between 30-125. Extreme skin breakout: In extreme skin breakout, an individual will foster countless enormous and difficult papules, pustules, knobs, or pimples. An individual may likewise have skin inflammation. The complete number of injuries is ordinarily north of 125. An individual's skin breakout stage might change after some time with their chemicals, feelings of anxiety, and another way-of-life factor all having an impact on the seriousness of their skin inflammation. Conditions like skin breakouts As indicated by the American Institute of Dermatology Affiliation (AAD), ailments that can cause or seem to be like skin breaks include: Polycystic ovary disorder (PCOS): a condition that influences the ovaries An individual with PCOS might encounter numerous hormonal side effects, including skin breakouts. Rosacea is a skin condition that results in redness or rashes on the face. It might also cause skin breakouts. Keratosis pilaris: a state of the skin that causes little, harsh knocks This normally happens on dry skin on the arms and thighs. Hidradenitis suppurativa is a condition that causes excruciating spots and scarring. These generally happen close to hair follicles that are close to perspiring organs, like in the armpits or on the upper thighs. Perioral dermatitis: This condition brings about little pimples around the mouth. These pimples might be red, dry, or seem to be a rash. Skin breakout happens when a pore becomes blocked up with dead skin cells, normal body oils, and microbes, including acne (C acne). At the point when these microorganisms enter and contaminate stopped pores, they cause aggravation and the development of skin break-out imperfections. The subsequent irritation can harm the construction of the follicle, permitting microbes, unsaturated fats, and lipids to pass into the encompassing skin. This can prompt more extensive aggravation, bunches of skin break-out sores, and more extreme skin break-outs, like cystic and nodular skin inflammation. When to see a specialist In instances of minor-to-direct skin breakouts, an individual might be expected to utilize home and OTC cures reliably for 2-3 months before they get results. More serious, provocative sorts of skin inflammation will generally take significantly longer to clear up. An individual ought to address a specialist or dermatologist if whiteheads, pimples, papules, or pustules are serious. Try not to answer OTC meds are extremely excruciating, have an extremely huge drain, a great deal of discharge, and cover a critical part of the face or body, causing profound misery. foster exceptionally near delicate regions, like the eyes or lips. Medicines Most dynamic fixings in OTC items are likewise accessible in original effectiveness medicines. A specialist might recommend these if an individual encounters serious skin breakout side effects. Dermatologists can treat huge, persevering sores. They can likewise eliminate those that don't respond to different types of treatment. An individual ought to continuously see a specialist or dermatologist about knobs and pimples because these require clinical consideration. Untreated knobs and growths, and those that have been picked or popped, can cause scarring. What is a hard pimple? Hard pimples are the result of dead skin cells or microorganisms getting under the skin. Hard pimples are profound, frequently enormous, and incidentally discharge-filled. They can be one of the most troublesome sorts of pimples to dispose of. How can I say whether my skin breakout is hormonal? Hormonal skin inflammation is not an alternate condition from skin inflammation. It is created because of changes in an individual's chemicals. An increase in testosterone can cause hormonal skin breakouts. For youths, hormonal skin breakout generally occurs in the "T-zone". This covers the temple, nose, and jawline. For adults aged 20 and over, hormonal skin breakout normally happens on the lower region of the face, like the jaw, jaw, and lower cheeks. An individual can work with a specialist to figure out what is causing the skin inflammation. How would I distinguish when my skin breaks out? There are different sorts of skin inflammation, and an individual might develop various types of spots depending on which type they have. For example, gentle skin inflammation is described by up to 30 clogged pores, whiteheads, and little papules or pustules. An individual with serious skin inflammation will have north of 100 pustules, papules, and growths and may find their skin inflammation difficult. An individual ought to visit a specialist or dermatologist to assist them with understanding the type and phase of skin inflammation they have. Outline There are a few sorts of skin inflammation. These can range from little knocks to serious growths. Skin breakouts can present as non-fiery flaws like pimples and whiteheads. This outcome is from the development of dead skin and oil in hair follicles and is most normal on the face, back, and chest. Assuming these blockages become tainted by microbes, they might become aggravated. Provocative types of skin inflammation can range from gentle knocks, like papules and pustules, to more serious structures, like knobs and blisters. Serious skin inflammation can adversely affect an individual's satisfaction. Be that as it may, an individual will want to oversee most types of skin inflammation at home with OTC cures.

Chapter 1

Nutritional deficiencies that lead to breakouts: what your body needs

Devouring particular kinds of food might assist with keeping the skin clear. A few food varieties have properties that decrease irritation and may assist with diminishing the presence of skin inflammation.

Nonetheless, skin inflammation can be because of a few factors, some inconsequential to eating less. On the off chance that an individual encounters skin inflammation, they might wish to talk with a specialist or dermatologist to track down the right answer for them.

Food to stay away from for more clear skin
On the off chance that an individual has worries about skin break out or just needs to ensure they are eating an eating regimen for solid skin, they might consider eating less of the accompanying food varieties.

Milk and dairy items
Restricted research proposes that milk and dairy items could add to skin conditions, like skin inflammation, in certain individuals.

A 2016 survey recommends a connection between high blood levels of the chemical IGF-1 and skin inflammation seriousness. IGF-1 communicates with adrenal organs, influencing chemicals in a way that adds to skin breakout. Since milk and other dairy items contain this chemical, it might make sense of a potential connection between dairy utilization and skin inflammation.

Notwithstanding IGF-1's effect on chemicals connected with skin breakout creation, different chemicals present in milk and dairy items might influence skin breakout both emphatically and adversely. The chemical estrogen, for instance, may diminish skin inflammation.

A few examinations of young ladies and young men have shown that polishing off dairy items, particularly skim milk, was related to having more skin breakouts. This might be because of diminished measures of estrogen in skim milk contrasted with entire milk.

Different parts of milk items may likewise impact skin inflammation. For instance, as per a more seasoned study, dairy contains the amino-corrosive leucine, which advances the development of sebum in skin cells.

Food sources with a high glycemic list
Research shows that eating regimens with a high glycemic list (GI) may add to skin breakout.

Food sources with a high GI raise glucose —
and subsequently insulin levels — quicker than
food sources with a lower GI.

Eating an eating routine with a high GI makes
the body produce more insulin. At the point
when the body has an overabundance of insulin,
it animates the development of androgen
chemicals and sebum in the skin, which can
prompt skin breakout.

Western weight control plans will quite often
incorporate food varieties with a high GI,
including:

refined grains
sweet grains
chips
treats
white bread
liquor
sweet drinks
food sources with added sugars

It is improbable that any single food on this rundown can cause skin to break out on the off chance that an individual eats it with some restraint. Be that as it may, following an eating regimen reliably high in a significant number of these food sources might assume a contributing part in creating skin breakouts.

Regardless of what B nutrient you're lacking, it can appear as a skin breakout the eight B nutrients, a lack in virtually every one of them can prompt a skin inflammation breakout. Since B12 is calming, a lack of this fundamental nutrient can exacerbate existing skin breakout without that extra line of safeguard. Biotin is normally hostile to contagious diseases, making an absence of this B nutrient reason and intensifying skin inflammation. Furthermore, B2 is fundamental for zinc retention, which is a mineral known to decrease the enlarging and redness brought about by skin breakout.

Does chocolate cause the skin to break out?

Episodically, many individuals accept that eating chocolate advances skin inflammation.

Be that as it may, a 2016 survey proposes there is no obvious proof between chocolate utilization and how much skin breakout an individual has. While certain individuals experience critical measures of skin inflammation after eating this food, others don't.

Concentrates on whether chocolate causes skin inflammation are uncertain. If there is a connection, it could be because of the milk and sugar content in certain kinds of chocolate.

Food sources that might assist with clear skin
To keep the skin at its best and assist with decreasing skin breakout, think about expanding the utilization of the accompanying food sources.

Greasy fish

Greasy fish is a wellspring of omega-3 fats, a fundamental piece of the eating routine with a few irrefutable positive well-being impacts.

A 2020 survey tracked down that consuming omega-3 unsaturated fats, like those tracked down in greasy fish, oversaw provocative skin conditions, including:

Skin inflammation
Skin ulcers
Psoriasis
Dermatitis
Furthermore, remembering omega-3s for the eating routine lessens the probability of creating skin malignant growth and may likewise diminish the impact specific medications have on the skin.

Broccoli
Broccoli and other cruciferous vegetables emphatically affect skin wellbeing. A recent report takes note that they contain sulforaphane,

which has cell reinforcement and calming properties.

Sulforaphane may likewise assist with forestalling untimely skin maturing by animating a few defensive cycles in skin cells and advancing immature microorganism reestablishment.

There isn't a lot of proof of the immediate impacts of broccoli on skin inflammation. In any case, one survey article found this vegetable and a few other plant food varieties contained low measures of leucine, an amino corrosive engaged with sebum creation.

At the point when the skin delivers an excess of sebum, it might leadTrusted Source to skin inflammation.

Soy
Soy might helpfully affect the skin.

A more established concentration requested that individuals consume 160 milligrams of a compound from soybeans called isoflavone consistently for a long time. The examination found members getting the isoflavone had fundamentally diminished skin break-out sores, or pimples, after treatment contrasted with the fake treatment bunch.

The treatment bunch additionally had diminished androgen chemical dihydrotestosterone (DHT) levels, which are connected with testosterone.

Elevated degrees of DHT and testosterone assume a part in expanding skin break-out improvement, as per a more established 2009 paper Confided in Source. In any case, specialists accept the chemical estrogen diminishes sebum creation, to some degree by repressing testosterone.

The isoflavones in soy are fundamentally like estrogen and can tie to estrogen receptors in the body. This might make sense of the connection between soy admission and estrogen-related well-being results, including skin flexibility, pigmentation, and vascularity.

There is some proof that consuming soy items might diminish kinks and increase how much collagen the body produces, which thus advances skin respectability.

Red grapes
Red grapes and red wine contain the compound resveratrol, which might have a few medical advantages.

One more seasoned in vitro concentrate on the microorganisms that cause skin break out found that resveratrol was to some degree harmful to skin inflammation microscopic organisms and attempted to repress them over the long haul. The specialists prescribed more examinations to explore resveratrol further as an expected treatment for skin inflammation.

A recent report found that resveratrol may valuably influence the skin in more than one way.

This substance might safeguard the skin by assisting it with remaining saturated and keeping it from losing heat.

Moreover, resveratrol may safeguard against UV harm. This might help safeguard against untimely maturing and different indications of sun harm, like kinks and liver spots.

Resveratrol likewise has a cell reinforcement impact that might assist with forestalling skin maturing, decreasing the presence of skin breakouts, and the improvement of skin issues. This incorporates skin malignant growths, like melanoma.

In any case, it is essential to take note that when an individual consumes resveratrol from dietary sources, they may not consider any significant impact to be that the centralization of resveratrol would be excessively low.

Chapter2

The role of digestive health in acne

As those with skin inflammation inclined skin know very well, there's no one-size-fits-all to deal with treating and forestalling breakouts. This can be staggeringly baffling and frequently individuals feel like they've attempted each skin-clearing chemical, cream, color, and treatment.

Propels in the examination of the stomach microbiome - the aggregate name for the trillions of microorganisms, or microorganisms, that live in your stomach - have empowered researchers to analyze the connection between stomach well-being and skin breakout more intently than at any other time. Their discoveries demonstrate we ought to shift focus over to the items in our supper plates, as opposed to our washroom cupboards, looking for a cure.

We address specialists, nutritionists, and microbiome specialists about the connection between stomach well-being and skin inflammation, pre- and probiotics, and which food sources are best for supporting your stomach well-being.

Does destroyed well-being and a defective stomach influence skin?
The personal connection between your skin - your body's biggest organ - and the microorganisms that live in your stomach is alluded to as the 'skin-stomach pivot'. Both are significant organs for keeping the body in a steady state and safeguarding against the attack of irresistible organic entities and the stomach microbiome. Frequently individuals with gastrointestinal illnesses, for example, provocative inside infection have related skin issues, which shows how firmly connected stomach wellbeing and skin wellbeing are.

While this relationship works the two different ways, the stomach microbiome is the key controller. Stomach microorganisms help to keep up with the digestive boundary, which limits bacterial side-effects, undigested proteins, and poisons from entering your blood dissemination and possibly arriving at the skin. The hindrance needs to open normally to let supplements through after dinner. Along these lines, it is typical for the stomach to 'spill'. However, when there is an irregularity among valuable and unsafe microscopic organisms that live in our stomach - called dysbiosis - the obstruction is debilitated.

While this relationship works the two different ways, the stomach microbiome is the key controller.

Dysbiosis can prompt aggravation and the arrival of provocative couriers called cytokines, which can add to the improvement of skin

inflammation. This irritation can likewise harm the covering of the stomach, permitting the microbe side effects to pass from the stomach through the circulatory system to the skin, where it can locally influence skin wellbeing, empowering the development of microscopic organisms that can set off Skin break out.
The results that are created by our stomach microorganisms likewise can change skin organisms, 'In a solid stomach, these side-effects could usefully affect our skin, while stomach dysbiosis and 'flawed stomach' could increment destructive side-effects into the flow and advance the excess of hurtful skin microbes like Cutibacterium acnes,'

Best items for treating skin inflammation and spots
The connection between stomach well-being and skin inflammation
Numerous provocative skin conditions have been straightforwardly connected to disturbances in stomach organisms, including skin breakout, rosacea, and dermatitis psoriasis. While

unfortunate stomach well-being is probably not going to be the sole reason for the advancement of skin break, stomach-related issues are more normal in those with skin inflammation than those without.

Skin breakout happens when an overabundance of skin lines within a hair follicle, impedes sebum from being discharged. This permits microorganisms to develop, getting a provocative reaction from your body's insusceptible framework. Strangely, roughly 70% of your body's resistant cells live in the stomach, where they are impacted by the stomach microbiome.

Certain valuable kinds of organisms seem to animate seriously quieting resistant cells, which could assist with directing the safe framework all through the body including the skin, While additional harmful microorganisms can prompt an invulnerable response, expanding aggravation both inside the stomach and possibly somewhere else in the body.

With regards to learning whether your stomach well-being could be a contributing element, it's down to experimentation, Assuming you have skin breakout, it very well may merit attempting to build your admission of prebiotic food sources - the food varieties that the 'great' stomach microorganisms like to eat - and taking a probiotic supplement (for example the actual microorganisms),

Skin break out: causes, triggers, and treatment
How might I further develop my stomach wellbeing for skin break out?
To improve your microbiome and readdress any lopsided characteristics between stomach microorganisms, you want dimension two-dimensional and foremost, center around adding 'great' microbes through a probiotic supplement. Search for an enhancement containing around 30 billion province framing

units (CFUs) and a mix of Lactobacillus and Bifidobacterium sp.

Then, you'll have to take care of those 'great' microscopic organisms with prebiotics, so they prosper and increase. ' Prebiotics incorporate matured food varieties like salted vegetables, fermented tea, kefir, crude vegetables - especially chicory root - leeks, onion, Jerusalem artichokes and asparagus, as well as crude garlic.

Enhancing with pre-and probiotics alone isn't sufficient. Center around eating an entire food varieties diet, high in brilliantly shaded products of the soil, sound wellsprings of fats, and great quality protein, Low glycaemic record consumes fewer calories have likewise shown enhancements in skin break out side effects, so keep away from sweet and handled food varieties and refined starches.

Fill your refrigerator with food varieties high in cell reinforcements including nutrients C and E, omega-3 unsaturated fats, retinoids (vitamin A), and follow metals like zinc. ' It's essential to take a comprehensive perspective and consider the eating routine as an entire and how this could connect with irritation in the skin.

Slick fish like salmon, mackerel, and herring are brilliant wellsprings of omega-3 unsaturated fats, which assume a 'huge part' in relieving provocative skin conditions, says Sana Khan, nourishment specialist and pioneer behind Avicenna Prosperity. Assuming you're a veggie lover or vegan, choose pecans, flaxseeds, chia seeds, and soybeans.

Top up with mitigating flavor flavors like dark pepper, ginger, cinnamon, clove, garlic, and cayenne. ' Being to a great extent plant-based in any place conceivable is a decent methodology with regards to boosting the degrees of cell reinforcements and mitigating synthetics in food sources.

In the meantime, creature-based items - especially dairy - have been displayed to set break out, as well as food varieties that are high in processed fats and sugars. This is because of the bevel cutting-getting edge glycation finished results (AGEs). ' The sugars are tied to underlying proteins in the skin and different tissues.

These are remembered to initiate the resistant framework, driving irritation. Also, food sources that have been cooked with dry warming cycles, for example, broiling and barbecuing are by and large high in receptive atoms and AGEs, so cooking strategies, for example, steaming are believed to blind

In lineup these speculations, studies are likewise beginning to propose that milk-rich weight control plans and an eating routine with a high glycaemic load (sugarloaf) bring about a more significant level of insulin and 'insulin-like development factor 1' (IGF-1), and this might be an immediate connection with demolishing skin break out. In adolescence, IGF-1 is raised because of expanding levels of chemicals and this might be one of the normal triggers for skin break out in these two situations. A few patients see enhancement for a veggie lover diet obviously, well-being are before rolling out tremendous improvements to your eating regimen.

Any dietary changes are thought to be on the foundation of a reasonable skincare system and conference with your primary care physician if skin inflammation is concerning you, not improving, or on the other hand assuming there is any tirelessness over the mildest spots

Chapter 3

Liver function and detoxification

There's a commonplace disarray that the liver is trustworthy only for taking care of alcohol, but nothing could be further from the real world! That is only one of the liver's many, many positions.

Close by filtering through harms - whether from alcohol, food, or a wide range of various things - your liver is one of the key organs related to keeping your skin sound.

If you want fewer breakouts and a sound shimmer, you should start by dealing with your liver prosperity.

How YOUR LIVER Prosperity Affects YOUR SKIN Prosperity

Many skin conditions - from skin break breakout mastitis to psoriasis - can be associated with awful liver capacity. A depleted liver can incite dry, troublesome skin, skin tone.

All that you eat, drink, and finish is taken care of by your liver, so keeping it despite how sound as conceivable might be huge.

You've no doubt heard that lamentable stomach prosperity can impact your skin. In light of everything, an improvement of toxic substances in the liver can in like manner achieve terrible skin discharges.

The liver is one of your body's basic removal organs. Any harm that you eat, drink, hold through your skin, or take in through your lungs should be filtered through by your liver. In various ways, your skin is a prompt impression of how beneficially that filtration cycle is working.

If your circulatory framework is over-trouble with harms - like food-engineered compounds, normal poisons, drugs, or alcohol — the results could show on your skin.

An obstructed liver is less prepared to isolate these toxins successfully, making them create. Thus, your body will endeavor to flush these toxic substances out in substitute ways, such as through your sweat. Right when those risky substances are expelled through your pores, they can upset and stir the skin. That is where breakouts can occur!

If you've ever done a purge, you could have experienced rashes or breakouts of skin irritation. This is much of the time in light of those terrible substances causing a provocative reaction.
Another component Related to the liver-skin break-out affiliation is fat. Another work that your liver does is to isolate the fat in your eating routine.

Exactly when your liver capacity is slow or inefficient, those fats will just float around in your course framework. Oftentimes, the oil-conveying organs in your skin (called the sebaceous organs) will endeavor to compensate for this extra fat and use them taking everything into account. Unfortunately, using this fat-dissolvable material to make sebum can prompt a large number of issues. These fats can disturb the ordinary oils on your skin since they will regularly contain provocative toxins.

The idea of fats in your dissemination framework will impact the idea of sebum on your skin. The thicker and more destructive the sebum, the practically 100% it will discourage your pores.

Expecting that your eating routine contains a high proportion of "horrible fats" - like those from burned food sources, chocolate, margarine, or other such food assortments - the impact on your skin will be essentially more limited. That suggests more breakouts!

3 Improvements TO Work on YOUR LIVER Prosperity

1. MILK Thistle

Milk thistle seeds contain areas of strength called silymarin. Silymarin is a critical disease counteraction specialist and conceivably the most impressive liver purifier in nature. It maintains and shields the liver by working on liver ability and detoxification. It works by limiting to the past the liver cells fighting off harms by discouraging their entry to the liver cell.

Clinical investigation has shown that this activity helps with supporting liver prosperity and reduces the bet of stretch damage to the liver.

Milk thistle's ability to speed up the detoxification cycle in the body can be hugely useful for steady skin break times liver is related to the rule of synthetics which can incite the improvement of skin irritation.

Exactly when certain synthetics assemble in the body, there may be an overproduction of sebum. This can provoke oil plugging up the pores in the skin, which can add to breakouts.

Milk thistle helps your liver with clearing these excess synthetic compounds off of the body. This is moreover one explanation it has for quite a while been used in Ayurvedic prescription as a blood purifier. It in like manner causes them to surprise disease counteraction specialists and quieting properties which could help with skin aggravation-related skin conditions.

2. DANDELION ROOT Concentrate
Standard prescription has long used dandelion root to chip away at liver prosperity and capacity.

Research recommends that dandelion root concentrate can help the movement of bile, which is major for the liver to do its various detoxification capacities.

Dandelion root tea is regularly recommended as a part of a liver filtering project and is even acknowledged to help with diminishing symptoms of liver contamination.

A new report showed that dandelion root could have hepatoprotective effects, while various assessments have found it reduced alcohol-provoked oxidative tension and besides facilitating -fat eating routine started non-alcoholic oily liver.

3. ARTICHOKE LEAF Concentrate

Artichoke leaf removal contains an enormous gathering of cell fortifications including cynarin and silymarin. Like milk thistle, this helps to safeguard the liver from cretaceous mischief and advance the improvement of new tissue.

Artichoke removal has in like manner been found to help the production of bile, which wipes out destructive toxic substances from the liver.

One survey including rodents showed that artichokes eliminated diminished liver mischief and further created disease counteraction specialist levels, achieving an overall improvement in liver capacity following an impelled medicine excess.

FocuStudiesindividuals in like manner show artichoke elimination deals with liver capacity in people with non-alcoholic oily liver disease, while a similar report showed taking artichoke separately regularly for quite a while achieved diminished liver bothering and less fat stores in the liver.

SUPPORTING YOUR LIVER

These are two or three of the various customary upgrades that can help with smoothing out your liver prosperity. Likewise, a superior liver will regularly mean better, more clear skin!

Every single one of those trimmings will maintain your liver, but they are extensively great when solidified into one upgrade.

Chapter 4

Hormonal balance

At the point when we consume some unacceptable data, we frequently think the "regular" move won't be essentially as compelling as a more cruel treatment like Accutane. False!

Brutal topicals, anti-conception medication pills, and drugs can obliterate the body from the back to front and are by all accounts not the only choice. Truly, these are old-school moves that don't consider the entire body as we do at NAC.

The American Foundation of Dermatology has found the beginning of grown-up skin breakout is turning out to be progressively normal in ladies in their 30s, 40s, and even 50s. Concentrates on show that up to half of ladies in their 20s and 25% of ladies in their 40s battle with skin breakouts set off by hormonal changes in the body.

Pregnancy, diet, stress, and menopause can cause a hormonal awkward nature setting off skin break out on the facial structure, jaw, or lower cheek. It can frequently seem red and excited causing some measure of agony.

The Connection Between Our Chemicals and Skin Break out

Before we get to the three best normal medicines for hormonal skin inflammation, how about we initially examine how chemicals trigger breakouts? Hold on for me briefly while we have a little science example!

Chemicals play a significant part in the improvement of skin breakouts. Albeit the specific instrument behind their strong impact is obscure, we in all actuality do realize that androgen chemicals gum up the follicle by setting off oil creation.

Androgens are the purported "male chemicals" and are available in guys and females. The testicles, ovaries, and the adrenal organs all produce androgens. The most notable androgens are testosterone and its breakdown item is dihydrotestosterone (DHT).

This is immensely significant because examination has shown there are androgen receptors in the foundation of the oil organ and in the cells that line the pores! Assuming there are elevated degrees of testosterone drifting in the body, they are profoundly equipped for restricting these receptors.

To lay it out, when these chemicals join the oil organs (also known as receptors) in the skin, they trigger the organ to create more oil as well as feed the microbes. Then, a kindled skin breakout injury is well en route to the outer layer of your skin.

Skin inflammation Sore

The key action item is that by bringing down androgen and testosterone levels in the body, the skin won't create as much skin break out or not produce ANY whatsoever.

So how does Estrogen play into this?

Estrogen and testosterone often behave like a seesaw. As one goes up the other goes down.

Hormonal skin breakout is a raised androgen/testosterone and low estrogen issue. It's anything but a raised estrogen issue. In this way, taking homegrown supplements that "block" estrogen, for example, Faint, will exacerbate your skin breakout and increase testosterone causing cystic breakouts. I don't suggest Fainting for hormonal skin break out thus.

So it's a good idea that assuming you lower androgen levels, the skin won't deliver as much oil — and your skin inflammation will get to the next level!

Momentum research demonstrates the way that Vitex can uphold solid chemical levels and assuage pre-feminine side effects. It can likewise be a successful normal hormonal skin inflammation treatment.

How does Vitex for Skin inflammation Function?
The Vitex spices follow up on the pituitary and nerve center organs by expanding luteinizing chemical (LH) creation and gently restraining the arrival of follicle-invigorating chemicals (FSH). This results in a change in the proportion of estrogen to progesterone, with an accent in progesterone. The capacity of the Vitex to increment progesterone levels is a roundabout impact.

Vitex itself isn't a chemical, but instead a spice that assists the body with adjusting normal estrogen and progesterone. By adjusting the estrogen, the androgens then, at that point, come into balance.

The most effective way to take Vitex for skin break out is by taking it first thing between 7-8 a.m. That is the point at which your pituitary and nerve center organs are dynamic to control female sex chemicals. You can hope to feel the full advantages of taking Vitex for skin inflammation inside 3-5 months.

Saw Palmetto

Saw Palmetto is a little palm with fan-molded leaves and strongly toothed stalks, local toward the southeastern US. Supplements produced using berries are utilized to diminish irritation and are found to diminish the take-up of testosterone in the body. These impacts are logically credited to regular enemies of androgenic impacts, which block the activities of testosterone in the body, which thus can assist with diminishing skin breakout breakouts for ladies and men.

While Saw Palmetto is principally advertised towards men, it tends to be utilized by females too! For ladies, this spice is suggested assuming periods are over 36 days separated or for females with indications of abundance testosterone like dim, coarse hair development on the upper lip, jaw, maritime or areola, PCOS conclusion, skin obscuring on the underarms, or overweight with little bosoms.

Saw Palmetto can likewise be utilized as a characteristic trade for Spironolactone when endorsed for skin inflammation since it is a characteristic androgen minimizer.

Saw Palmetto
Omega-3 Unsaturated fats

Omega 3 unsaturated fats EPA and DHA have likewise been demonstrated to be a successful hormonal skin inflammation treatment. In addition to the fact that these fundamental unsaturated fats calm your body's fiery reaction to overabundant sebum and microbes, however, they likewise assist with adjusting skin break-causing chemicals like testosterone and androgen.

Taking Clove Slope SkinOmega-3 as well as eating food varieties high in Omega 3's can be a powerful hormonal skin inflammation treatment.

SkinOmega-3
2. Hormonal Skin break out Diet
In 1984, the main review was led in Finland that showed an eating routine chemical association.

Decline your admission of immersed fat:

In 1984, the principal study was led in Finland that showed an eating routine chemical association. In one six-week study, Dr. Esa Hamalainen and her group showed that changing from an eating regimen high in immersed fat to one with 38% not so much fat but rather more polyunsaturated fats (nuts, seeds, fish, green growth, mixed greens) caused a huge decrease in androstenedione (forerunner to testosterone) and testosterone.

Increment fiber utilization:

Indeed, eating fiber can assist with clearing your skin! One review distributed in the American Diary of Clinical Sustenance found that counting calories high in refined carbs brought about a higher frequency of skin breakouts. Research shows that a high-fiber diet can diminish blood testosterone, DHT, and DHEA — androgens that trigger hormonal skin inflammation.

In America, the typical everyday utilization of fiber is 13 grams. The suggested day to day measurements are 25 grams for ladies and 38 grams for men. So changing from white cuts of bread, rice, and pasta to high-fiber, entire wheat food sources can assist with diminishing the seriousness of skin break out.

Avoid cow's dairy (particularly cow's milk):

Research demonstrates the way that dairy can make skin break out due to elevated degrees of iodine. Entire milk itself doesn't normally contain iodine, ranchers give their cows iodine-braced feed to forestall disease. They additionally use iodine answers for disinfecting cow udders and draining gear. Subsequently, the iodine gets into the actual milk.

As per research distributed in the Diary of the American Foundation of Dermatology drinking dairy - explicitly, low-fat/skim milk — is a lot higher in teens who have skin break out. More secure choices are goat and sheep milk.

Increment basic food varieties and diminishing acidic food varieties:

Meat-based proteins, espresso, liquor, sugar, and handled grains - all food varieties that are a major piece of the commonplace American eating routine — are corrosive framing in the framework. This prompts a condition called acidosis. Acidosis is the specialized term for

over-fermentation. The fundamental side effect
of acidosis is weakness.

pixels Andres Ayrton
Different side effects incorporate loss of
excitement forever, loss of sex drive, unfortunate
rest quality, despondency, and tiring rapidly both
intellectually and truly. High-level stage side
effects of acidosis incorporate aversion to colds,
low circulatory strain, hypo or hyperthyroidism,
and low glucose.

These side effects are caused in light of the fact
that the fundamental minerals that are expected
to feed the sensory system, like calcium,
magnesium, and potassium, are exactly the same
minerals that the body uses to kill acids!

Concentrates on showing that soluble food
sources like organic products, vegetables, and
entire grains assist with killing these acids. By
simply eating all the new natural products,
vegetables, and entire grains in supplant of meat,
sugar, and other handled food sources, you won't

accept how astonished you feel in only a couple of days!

3. Stress Decreases indeed, it influences our chemicals!
Nowadays, beginning from kindergarten, the strain is on. We as a whole encounter it and make an honest effort to diminish it.

Also, assuming you've seen additional pimples during seasons of pressure, you're in good company. Research shows there's a clear connection between stress and skin inflammation breakouts.

Stress enacts the adrenal organs to create additional androgen chemicals which in the long run brings about kindled skin break out breakouts in skin inflammation inclined skin. These additional chemicals animate the sebaceous organs in the skin and trigger a breakout.

The pressure chemical association is to a greater degree an issue for ladies as opposed to it for men since they produce a large portion of their male chemicals (androgens) in their adrenal organs. Men, then again, produce a large portion of their male chemicals in the testicles and just a tiny sum in the adrenal organs.

Adrenal Organ
Men's essential chemical is testosterone so when they get pushed and the body delivers additional testosterone, it doesn't have as large of an effect as it accomplishes for ladies. Since ladies produce around one-10th of as much testosterone as men, an unexpected flood of extra testosterone can essentially affect the body — and the skin.

Furthermore, stress additionally causes elevated degrees of causticity. Eating more soluble food varieties kills these acids while likewise decreasing cortisol levels.

To safeguard our adrenal organs from this flood of androgens (testosterone), we need to safeguard them! The Adrenal Pressure Recipe is one of the most straightforward ways of keeping that spike of androgens from influencing our skin and setting off a pressure breakout.

Try not to Misjudge Nature's Recuperating Power.

Chapter 5

Inflammation

performed by an expert, or they could harm the pores and lead to more skin inflammation.

HOME Solutions for Skin Break out AND HOW TO Utilize THEM

Beneath, we examine the best home solutions for skin break out, what the examination says, and way of life changes that can help.

On the off chance that an individual is keen on attempting specific skin cures, it is smart to chat with a dermatologist before applying the skin cure straightforwardly to the skin or do a fix test first, which comprises of putting a modest quantity of the skin treatment on the wrist or hand to test for skin responses.

1. Tea tree oil
Tea tree oil is a characteristic antibacterial and calming, and that implies that it could kill P. acnes, the microscopic organisms that cause skin break out.

Tea tree oil's calming properties imply that it can likewise assist with decreasing the expansion and redness of pimples.

A 2019 survey study took a gander at the current proof of tea tree oil and skin breakout. The scientists found that tea tree oil items can diminish the quantity of skin break-out bruises in individuals due to tea trees' antimicrobial capacities.

This equivalent survey likewise noted research showing the complete number of skin breakout injuries of study members was diminished from 23.7 to 10.7 following two months of utilizing tea tree oil facial items.
The most effective method to utilize tea tree oil

Individuals can apply tea tree concentrate to their skin and break out in creams, gels, or medicinal ointments. Nonetheless, a 2016 survey article brings up that tea tree oil can cause hypersensitive responses in certain people, and recommends individuals use tea tree oil items under 5% confided in Source fixation to keep away from skin bothering.

Even though exploration proposes that natural ointments might have some medical advantages, it is vital to recall that the Food and Medication Organization (FDA) doesn't screen or control the virtue or nature of these. An individual ought to converse with a medical care proficient before utilizing medicinal ointments, and they ought to make certain to investigate the nature of a brand's items. An individual ought to constantly do a fixed test before attempting another natural balm.

2. Jojoba oil
Jojoba oil is a characteristic, waxy substance removed from the seeds of the jojoba bush.

The waxy substances in jojoba oil might assist with fixing harmed skin, which may likewise assist with accelerating wound mending, including skin break-out sores.

A portion of the mixtures in jojoba oil could assist with lessening skin irritation, which might decrease redness and expand around pimples, whiteheads, and other excited sores.

In a recent report, scientists gave 133 individuals earth facial coverings that contained jojoba oil. Following a month and a half of utilizing the veils a few times each week, individuals revealed a 54% improvement in skin breakout.

Instructions to utilize jojoba oil
Take a stab at blending jojoba rejuvenating ointment with a gel, cream, or earth facial covering and apply it to skin inflammation. In any case, place a couple of drops of jojoba oil on a cotton cushion and rub this tenderly over skin break-out wounds.

3. Aloe vera

Aloe vera is a characteristic antibacterial and mitigating, meaning it might lessen the presence of skin inflammation and forestall skin breakout breakouts.

Aloe vera contains sugar atoms, amino acids, and zinc, making it an amazing skin lotion and protectant. It is particularly reasonable for individuals who get dry skin from other enemies of skin break-out items.

In a recent report, specialists established that the number of knocks, sores, and dry skin was brought down while utilizing aloe vera joined with ultrasound and delicate veil applications.

Step-by-step instructions to utilize aloe vera gel
An individual ought to clean skin inflammation injuries and afterward apply a slim layer of cream or gel two times day to day after purifying with cleanser.

4. Honey

For millennia, honey has treated skin conditions since it contains numerous cell reinforcements that can assist with clearing stopped-up pores.

In any case, while there is proof that honey makes explicit antimicrobial impacts, a 2016 survey believed Source didn't find areas of strength for honey's impact on skin breakout explicitly.

The most effective method to utilize honey Utilizing a perfect finger or cotton cushion, rub some honey into the pimples. In any case, add honey to a face or body veil.

5. Zinc

With its mitigating properties, zinc is in many cases promoted as a strategy to decrease skin break-out sores and redness.

As indicated by a 2021 article, research is clashing on zinc's viability. Nonetheless, an individual can expect improved results while applying the enhancement straightforwardly to the skin. The explanation is that when taken orally, a portion of the enhancement gets separated in the absorption cycle and may lose viability en route.

Step-by-step instructions to utilize zinc
Individuals can apply zinc topically onto the skin or take it in a supplement structure.

6. Green tea
Green tea contains high centralizations of a gathering of polyphenol cell reinforcements called catechins.

Certain individuals with skin breakouts have an excessive amount of sebum, or regular body oils, in their pores and insufficient cell reinforcements. Cancer prevention agents assist the body with separating synthetics and side effects that can harm sound cells.

Green tea additionally contains intensifies that might serve to:

decrease the skin's sebum creation

decrease P. acnes

decrease aggravation

The most effective method to utilize green tea

An individual can either drink green tea or put green tea extricate on their skin, however, scientists say the current proof is restricted.

Nonetheless, one 2017 review, found a 79-89 % trusted Source decrease in whiteheads and clogged pores after utilizing a polyphenol green tea removed for a considerable length of time.

Individuals can find green tea in most food stores. Green tea separately is more difficult to see as yet accessible from some well-being stores or on the web.

7. Echinacea

Echinacea, otherwise called purple coneflower, may contain intensifiers that help obliterate infections and microscopic organisms, including P. acnes.

Many individuals accept that echinacea can help the insusceptible framework and decrease irritation to ward off or forestall contaminations, including colds and influenza. While there is some proof that echinacea can assist with halting the spread of P. acnes and the opposite irritation brought about by microscopic organisms, flow research is insignificant.

The most effective method to utilize echinacea Individuals can apply echinacea creams to regions with skin inflammation sores or take echinacea supplements. Echinacea items are accessible from wellbeing stores or online as creams or enhancements.

8. Rosemary
Rosemary concentrates, or Rosmarinus officinalis contain synthetics and mixtures with cell reinforcement, antibacterial, and calming properties.

Further examination is expected to gauge its viability. Nonetheless, a 2016 exploration article recommended that rosemary concentrate can lessen irritation from the skin inflammation causing microscopic organisms P. acnes.

9. Cleansed honey bee toxin
Even though it's not broadly accessible, decontaminated honey bee toxin contains antibacterial properties.

In a recent report, individuals who applied a gel containing refined honey bee toxin to their face for a long time saw a decrease in gentle to direct skin breakout sores.

However more examination is required, decontaminated honey bee toxin might be a helpful future fixing in skin break out prescription.

10. Coconut oil
Like a few other normal cures recorded, coconut oil contains calming and antibacterial mixtures.

These properties imply that coconut oil might assist with destroying skin break-causing microbes and decrease the redness and enlarging of pimples. Because of its alleviating and saturating effectsTrusted Source, coconut oil might assist with accelerating the mending of open skin breakout injuries. Nonetheless, centered research around coconut oil as a skin breakout obstacle is deficient.

The most effective method to utilize coconut oil Take a stab at scouring unadulterated, virgin coconut oil straightforwardly into the area with skin inflammation. Search for coconut oil in the normal food varieties part of supermarkets or on the web.

Way of life changes for skin break out Alongside home cures, explicit way-of-life changes can capably affect keeping the body solid, making the skin less sleek, and decreasing skin break-out eruptions.

11. Try not to contact pimples
It tends to be exceptionally enticing, however contacting skin breakout injuries will bother the skin, may aggravate the pimple, and can spread pimples to different regions.

Contacting, scouring, crushing, or popping skin inflammation wounds can likewise bring more microbes into the injury, creating additional contamination. Crunching a pimple can drive microorganisms and garbage further into the skin, so the spot might return more terrible than it was previously.

Talk with a specialist about huge injuries or those profound under the skin to figure out how to securely treat them.

12. Picking the right chemical
Numerous standard cleansers have a causticity or pH, that is excessively high and can bother the skin, exacerbating skin breakout.

Pick gentle cleaning agents, flushes, and washes to decrease the gamble of skin inflammation eruptions and allow wounds to recuperate.

13. Utilizing without oil skincare
Oil-based or oily items can hinder pores, expanding the gamble of stopping and developing skin inflammation injuries.

Search for skincare items and beauty care products named "without oil" or "noncomedogenic," which contain fixings that permit pores to relax.

14. Remaining hydrated
At the point when the skin is dry, it can become disturbed or harmed, which can exacerbate skin inflammation. Remaining hydrated likewise guarantees new skin cells grow accurately as wounds mend.

There is no standard day-to-day suggested water admission because every individual's water needs shift contingent on age, how dynamic they are, temperature, and any ailments.

Putting forth a concentrated attempt to hydrate during the day is a decent beginning stage.

15. Lessening pressure
The American Foundation of Dermatology records pressure as a potential reason for skin break-out eruptions.

Stress makes levels of the chemical androgen increment. Androgen animates hair follicles and oil organs in pores, expanding the gamble of skin breakout.

Ways to oversee pressure include:

conversing with family, companions, a specialist, or other strong individuals
getting sufficient rest
eating a fortifying, adjusted diet
practicing routinely
restricting liquor and caffeine utilization

rehearsing profound breathing, yoga, care, or
reflection
Clinical medicines for skin breakout
There are numerous clinical treatment choices
for skin break out, and many are profoundly
compelling, however, they can c, cause
incidental effects and may not be appropriate for
everybody.

Individuals can talk with a specialist about
whether utilizing drugs or therapeutic creams is
ideal for them, basically on the off chance that
home cures have not worked.

Individuals might need to chat with their PCP in
the event bruises are:

extremely difficult
frequently contaminated
profound under the skin
not answering home treatment
covering an enormous area of skin
causing profound pain

There are times when an individual ought to see a specialist if they have skin break out in light of the hidden causes.

Chapter 6

How to get rid of acne scars

From the past parts, you ought to have understood what caused your skin inflammation, knowing the reason for your skin inflammation, helps the scar purifying technique to be quick and simple.

Kinds of Skin inflammation Scar

The kinds of skin inflammation scars are as per the following:
Atrophic scars: These are skin breakouts that induce pinprick scars: These are little scars that look like pinpricks.
Car scars: Scars that show up as bigger spaces with clear edges.
Moving scars: These present as muddled edges, giving the skin an undulating appearance.

Hypertrophic scars: A raised scar remains when the skin delivers such a large number of fibroblasts while mending a skin break out trophic scars, these are typically greater than the skin breakout pigmentation and tingling.
The uplifting news is you can initially figure out how to treat skin inflammation scars at home before clinical medications It may, in the experience of Skin break, looking for clinical help would be ideal.

What Causes Skin to Break out Scars?
Before we get into how to eliminate skin breakouts, we should comprehend the main driver of skin inflammation. Skin inflammation causes scars when it enters the skin so profoundly that the hidden tissue is harmed. The body attempts to fix the harm as the skin inflammation mends. Right now, the body produces collagen. Excessively little or a lot of collagen prompts scarringIfIn thdoesn't't deliver sufficient collagen, you will see discouraged skin break-out scars after the skin inflammation mends. Nonetheless, if your body delivers an

excess of collagen, you will foster a raised skin break-out scar. By and large, it is feasible to eliminate skin break-out scars.

Side effects of Skin inflammation Scars
You will see different scarring depending upon the sort of skin break-out, you encounter, like whiteheads, pimples, growths, and so on., what's more, where it showed up. If you notice any of these side effects, you will want to in like manner settle on a treatment decision. The side effects are as per the following:

Discouraged scarring generally happens on the face. This incorporates rolling, ice pick, or car scars.
Icepick scars are noticeable on the temple and upper cheeks.
Moving scars can be found on the lower cheeks and jaw.
Boxing scars are likewise generally found on the jaw and lower cheeks.

Raised scars are the aftereffect of the overabundance of collagen delivered by the body. These scars are typically tracked down on the shoulders, chest, facial structure, and back. They are likewise excruciating or bothersome. Now that we know the kinds of skin break-out scars and their side effects, we should figure out how to eliminate skin inflammation scars normally.

Eliminate Skin inflammation Scars Normally At Home

Recognizing various kinds of skin break-out scarring is significant. Assuming that the main driver is perceived, we can pick the right treatment technique. Scarring frequently drives us to feel underconfident in our appearance. Be that as it may, imagine a scenario where there were simple skin inflammation scar cures we could do comfortably. Indeed, you can figure out how to eliminate pimple checks normally at home. If you are considering how to eliminate skin break-out scars normally, it is conceivable with a couple of home cures.

Before you head to the specialist, attempt these home solutions for skin inflammation scars:

1) Lemon
You can utilize lemon to blur skin and break out scars. Right off the bat, it contains L-ascorbic acid, which helps fabricate harmed cells in the skin. Furthermore, citrus extract attempts to eliminate dead skin cells. Thirdly, it likewise contains Alpha-hydroxy corrosive, which goes about as a blanching fixing, consequently blurring scars.

You can apply it straightforwardly on your skin if you are not going out in the sun. On the other hand, you might utilize a lemon facial covering.

2) Egg Whites
Eggs are an extraordinary wellspring of protein that is great for your overall well-being. Nonetheless, you can utilize the whites of the egg to treat scarring.

Utilize a cotton ball to plunge the white of the egg and apply it all over. After it dries, you can flush it off your skin. You might lay down with it on and wash it toward the beginning of the day.

3) Aloe Vera Gel
Aloe Vera is genuinely simple to source and has lots of therapeutic worth.

Cut a piece of the aloe vera leaf and strip the external part. Utilize the new gel straightforwardly on your skin. Besides the fact that it helps blur the scars, it additionally saturates your face. Knead it on and leave it for 30 minutes before washing it off.

4) Olive Oil
Olive oil contains cancer prevention agents that assist with recuperating skin, accordingly treating your scars simultaneously.

You should simply dunk a cotton ball in olive oil and straightforwardly apply it to your face. Rub a little olive oil onto your face consistently for the best impact.

5) Sandalwood
Sandalwood is usually utilized in Indian families to treat a bunch of skin issues.

Blend some sandalwood powder with water and make a glue. Apply the glue to the impacted region of your skin. Following 15-20 minutes, you can wash it off.
6) Tomato Cuts or Mash
Tomato contains two essential fixings; Vitamin An and Carotenes. Wealthy in cell reinforcements, tomato is ideal for blurring scars.

You can apply tomato cuts or mash on your skin to help mend scarring.

7) Baking Pop
Baking Soft drink has dying properties which is the reason they turn out superb for scarring treatment.

You essentially have to make glue from 2-3
spoons of baking pop and water and apply it on
your skin for a couple of moments.

8) Potato Cuts
Potatoes are plentiful in supplements like
Nutrients C and B6, flavonoids, and potassium.

Cut a couple of cuts of potatoes and rub them on
your skin day to day. Before long, the scarring
will blur. This assists with reducing redness,
tingling, and irritation of the skin.

9) Honey
Honey, a characteristic cream can assist with
recuperating your skin.

Tenderly back-rub crude honey onto the
impacted region of your skin consistently. You
can add a couple of drops of lemon juice to
honey to work on the possibilities of mending.

10) Cucumber

Cucumber has skin-fixing and saturating abilities, which are valuable for treating skin inflammation scars.

Cut a cucumber and put the cuts all over for around 20-30 minutes. Then, at that point, clean up. You can do this 3-5 times each week.

11) Turmeric Powder
Turmeric assists with lighting up the skin and gives it an even tone.

You can make a simple Do-It-Yourself veil by blending turmeric and water to make glue. Apply it all over and let it dry. After it dries totally, wash it off with tepid water. It will likewise assist with diminishing irritation.
18) Besan
Besan treats skin inflammation scars as it sheds the skin, eliminates soil and dead skin cells, and eases up the skin.

You can scowl pack by blending besan with water to make a glue. Apply it all over for 15 minutes before washing it off. Get done with a cream.

19) Apple juice vinegar

Apple juice vinegar splashes over the top oil and normally sheds the skin. It can likewise diminish the redness of skin inflammation and make them more modest. Dunk a cotton ball in apple juice vinegar and apply it all over. Following 20 minutes, wash it off with cool water.

20) Castor Oil

Castor oil attempts to fix harmed skin and advance the development of new skin cells. It additionally helps decline hyperpigmentation and decreases skin break-out scars. Utilize the cotton ball technique to apply castor oil onto your face for a couple of moments. Nonetheless, as it has a thick consistency, you should ensure you wash it off appropriately.

As may be obvious, there are a lot of manners by which we can figure out how to eliminate skin break-out scars normally. In any case, before figuring out how to treat skin break-out scars at home, we should find out about a few preventive tips for skin breakout

Preventive Tips For Skin Break And Pimple Scars

Not all are sufficiently lucky to be honored with impeccable skin. A few of us get skin inflammation sensibly frequently. It's adequately baffling to manage the aggravation of skin inflammation, not to mention it leaving flaws on our skin. In any case, there are things that we can do to keep it from leaving scars. There are ways of treating skin break-out scars at home by keeping them from showing up in any case. These include:

Utilize a non-comedogenic face wash two times per day.
Never lie down with your cosmetics on. Wash it off before getting into bed.
By no means would it be advisable for you to pop your pimples.

Continuously apply sunscreen, regardless of whether you're not heading outside. It additionally shields your skin from the blue light of gadgets.
Eat a decent eating routine and hydrate consistently.
Additionally Read: Pimples In the Wake of Shaving ~ 7 Science-Supported Activities

How Might I Diminish My Gamble of Skin Breakout Out Scars?
There are various manners by which you can decrease your possibility of getting skin break-out scars. Right off the bat, consistently wear sunscreen. Besides, never pick at your pimples, as this increases aggravation. Thirdly, treat your skin inflammation right away and not sit tight for it to deteriorate. Ultimately, abstain from smoking, as tobacco builds the gamble of skin scarring.

If you have any desire to know how to eliminate skin inflammation scars normally, you can follow the above techniques. Ultimately, on the off chance that no preventive measure or home cure works, look for proficient assistance and visit a dermatologist.

When to Look for Clinical Assistance?
Skin break-out scars are a typical peculiarity. In any case, passing on it to recuperate all alone may not be the best thing to do. If you know how to eliminate skin reak-out scars normally, attempt home cures. You might attempt home cures however don't self-sedate. In any case, if you experience serious skin breakouts, visiting your dermatologist quickly is ideal.

12) Coconut Oil
Coconut oil is an extraordinary lotion with mending capacities.

Take a couple of drops of coconut oil on your palm and rub it into your skin. You want not to wash this off. Be that as it may, on the off chance that you could do without the surface, you might wash it off following 30 minutes.

13) Chilled green tea

Green tea ends up containing an elevated degree of cell reinforcements, which battle free extremists that harm your skin. It likewise has germicide characteristics that dispense with skin break-causing microorganisms.

To involve it in your skincare schedule, you want to soak a green tea pack in warm water. In the wake of eliminating the sack, empty the fluid into a plate and put it in the cooler. Utilize each ice block in turn to rub all over.

14) Green coconut water

Coconut water contains skin break out taking out cytokinins and cell reinforcements. It likewise fixes drooping skin.

Get a new green coconut and cut it open. Empty out the water into a bowl. Rather than drinking it, utilize a cotton ball to wipe it all over. Then clean up with tepid water. Step-by-step instructions to utilize

15) Fenugreek (methi)

As fenugreek has disinfectant and calming properties, it assists with taking out the development of skin breakouts and skin contaminations.

Douse a modest bunch worth of methi seeds for the time being in a bowl of water. Make a fine glue of the seeds and add a couple of drops of rosewater. Utilize a warm towel all over to open pores before you apply the glue all over. After it evaporates, clean up with cold water.

16) Tea tree oil

Tree tea oil is both disinfectant and antibacterial, forestalling skin contamination and mending wounds.

Take a couple of drops of tea tree oil in your palm and back-rub it into the impacted region. Following 10 minutes, plunge a cotton ball into some tepid water and eliminate the overabundance of oil from your face.

17) Yogurt and honey veil
Yogurt contains a substance called alpha
hydroxy acids that work to limit the redness of
skin breakouts and different imperfections on
your skin.

In the first place, blend 2 tablespoons of yogurt
with 1 tablespoon of honey. Then, at that point,
apply the cover to your face and flush with tepid
water following 10 minutes.